Reduce Risks Around Your Home

A Preparedness Guide!

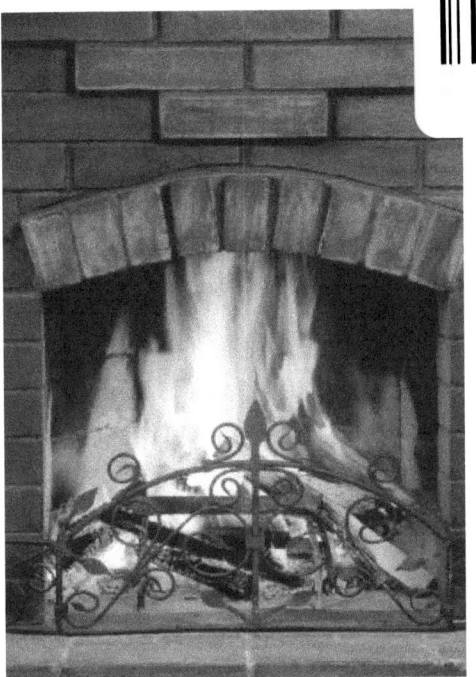

Survival and Prepping Series

M. Usman

Mendon Cottage Books

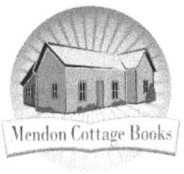

JD-Biz Publishing

Disclaimer

The information is this book is provided for informational purposes only. It is not intended to be used and medical advice or a substitute for proper medical treatment by a qualified health care provider. The information is believed to be accurate as presented based on research by the author.

The contents have not been evaluated by the U.S. Food and Drug Administration or any other Government or Health Organization and the contents in this book are not to be used to treat cure or prevent disease.

The author or publisher is not responsible for the use or safety of any diet, procedure or treatment mentioned in this book. The author or publisher is not responsible for errors or omissions that may exist.

Warning

The Book is for informational purposes only and before taking on any diet, treatment or medical procedure, it is recommended to consult with your primary health care provider.

Our books are available at
1. Amazon.com
2. Barnes and Noble
3. Itunes
4. Kobo
5. Smashwords
6. Google Play Books

Table of Contents

Preface

In life, there are a lot of things that have the potential to destroy us in the blink of an eye. We could talk of lighting, earthquakes, tsunamis, and more. While many are of the belief that being on the road increases the chances, we have to realize that danger also awaits us everywhere, even in our homes. From poisoning to house fires, the list is really long.

But, it is not supposed to be that way. Home is supposed to be where you can rest and enjoy some quality time with the family. The good thing is you have the liberty to secure your home as much as you want.

In this book, you will discover how you can reduce some accidents likely to occur in your home. This is not an assurance that by following the advice given in this book, you will never have accidents in your house. Think of it as wearing a seatbelt when in a car - it does not mean you will survive if an accident is to happen. Rather, you only increase your chances of surviving.

Enjoy the reading.

Chapter # 1: Reducing the Risk of Fire

Without fire, the human race would probably have had a difficult time surviving, even though we only use it for cooking and heating. But at the same time, we have to agree that the same fire that has helped us survive can turn deadly at times. In America, on average, 7 people die on a daily basis from fires and 36 more are treated for injuries.

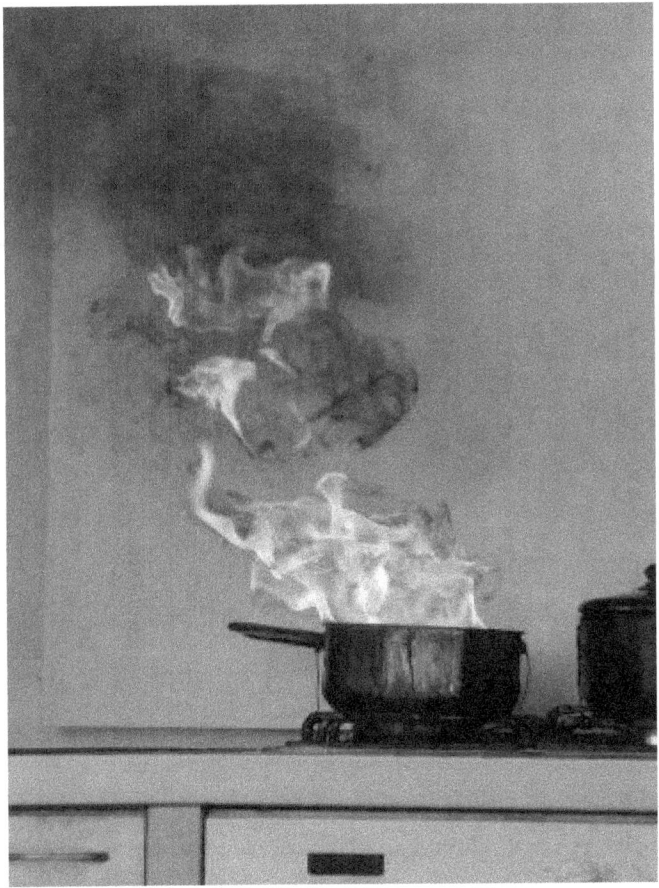

Heaters, holiday lights, defective appliances, lighters, and many other things pose the risk of a fire. It only takes seconds for it to start, and in minutes it becomes impossible to see your way out, because of the black smoke that fills the house.

So it makes a lot of sense to take measures that will reduce the risk of a fire starting in your house. Here are some things you can do:

- ***Do Not Overload Power Outlets***: Having a number of electrical appliances connected to the same power outlet multiplies the risk of a fire. What makes it even worse is that these might be left unattended. As a solution, hire a professional to install more outlets. What you will lose in money is minimal if compared to what will be destroyed when a fire starts.

- ***Turn Off Holiday Lights When Away***: These are one of the biggest fire starters during the holidays. The problem lies in the fact that these are reused several times and never inspected for damage during installation. Adding salt to the wound is that we leave them on, as we are asleep or away.

- ***Keep Flammable Things Away from Heat Sources***: This includes keeping such things as tea towels, curtains, clothes, or anything that can easily catch fire away from a heat source (stove, candle etc.). It is quite shocking how people always overlook this.

- ***Unplug Electrical Appliances***: It is recommended that you unplug all electrical appliances when going away or to sleep, yet many ignore this. If you are among them, try to at least turn off the appliances from the socket. And always double check to ensure that heating appliances (burners, heaters etc.) are off.

- ***Build Walls with Fire Resistant Material***: Using such materials as bricks or concrete will help make your walls resistant to fire.

- ***Keep Flammable Stuff Away from Children***: This includes lighters, matches, fuel, candles, etc.

- ***Be Careful With Space Heaters***: These provide a great way of keeping warm when it is cold, but time and again, we misuse them resulting in house fires. So if you decide to use one of these, keep it away from things that can easily catch fire (bed, curtains, clothes etc.).

- ***Do Not Smoke in Bed***: You will likely fall asleep if you smoke in bed and such incidences are well known for starting fires. The same is true if you smoke when drunk or tired – so try to avoid this. Additionally, have ashtrays if you allow smoking in your house.

- ***Have a Fire Blanke***t: Have this and make sure you know how to use it. For example, if fire starts in a pan while cooking, a fire blanket is the best way to put it out.

- ***Clean Chimneys***: About 50% of home fires are chimney fires. To avoid this, it is recommended that you clean yours at least twice a year.

- ***Install Smoke Alarms***: Since no amount of prevention will guarantee that a fire will not start in your house, it is recommended to install fire alarms in every room. You should also try to make sure that they work by testing them at least once a month. Additionally, you should change the batteries once every year.

- ***Have Extinguishers***: You should also have fire extinguishers and they should always be charged.

- ***Practice Fire Drills***: Knowing how to act in the moment will save you, so have fire drills at least once every year. This is especially helpful if you have kids or the elderly in the house.

Chapter # 2: Minimize the Risk of Falling

Anyone is at a risk of falling. As a matter of fact, no one can admit to having never fallen in his or her life. However, older people are the ones at the highest risk. Looking at the statistics, in U.S.A alone, 1 out of 3 adults fall annually. And in every 29 minutes, an adult dies as a result of falling. This can be attributed to sight problems, medication, and perhaps weak muscles among other reasons.

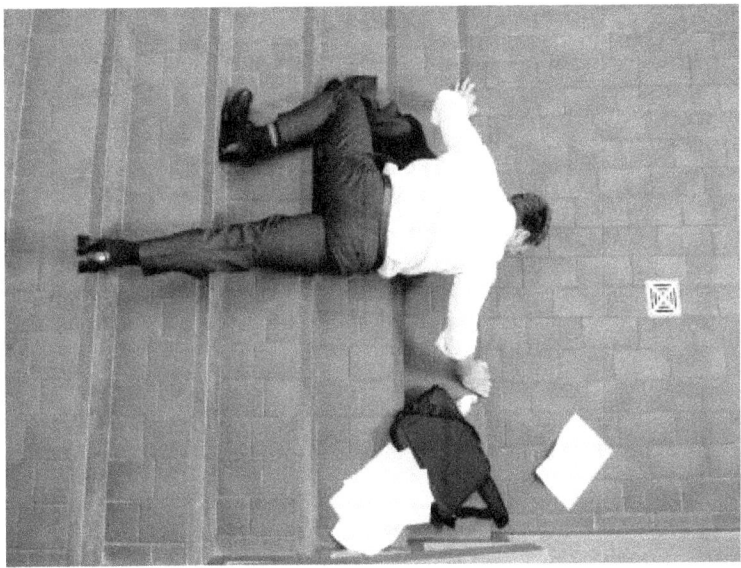

Falling also happens to be the leading cause of injury in older people. Here are some steps you can take to reduce this risk in your house:

- **Secure Rugs**: Rugs that are loose are disasters waiting to happen. As a solution, you can use tape to secure such rugs. However, the best solution is to remove them completely.

- **Clear Walkways**: Remove boxes, buckets, tables, electrical cords and anything that might trip a person. If you cannot remove them, secure them down.

- ***Make Items Accessible***: There are some things that are needed frequently for use. Consider putting these somewhere accessible, as someone might be tempted to use a stool for reaching these items.

- ***Clean Spills***: Spilling water or food on the floor is something inevitable. But, it is advisable to clean this immediately because someone might fall as a result.

- ***Provide Enough Illumination***: You should have enough light in the house, as there could be something on the floor that might cause someone to fall. You should never forget the stairs as this is where most falls occur.

- ***Install Hand Rails***: You should also have handrails on both sides of stairs, as this could help someone go up and down safely.

- ***Install Grab Bars***: You should have these in the shower, bathtub, and near the toilet.

- ***Wear Proper Shoes***: Your shoes should properly fit and preferably, be flat. High heels are not recommended. In addition, you should never try to walk with socks only.

- ***Exercise***: Simply having some exercise now and then will reduce your chances of falling, as it will make your muscles strong. The exercises does not need to be strenuous - even dancing would do.

- ***Talk to a Doctor***: If you have had a fall recently, the likelihood of having another one is high. In some situations, this could be a result of medication or a medical condition. The doctor will help you identify the cause and recommend ways of reducing the chances of it happening again.

- ***Follow Proper Nutrition***: Having a good diet will go a long way in reducing your chances of falling. Some foods, for example, will boost your energy, vision, and strengthen muscles.

Chapter # 3: Prevent Poisoning

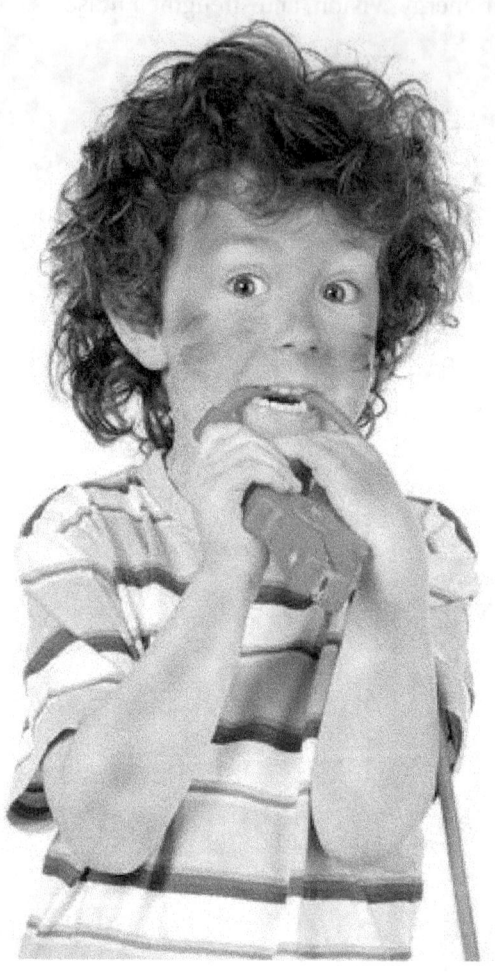

As infants start to walk and explore the house, extra care must be taken to prevent accidents. Actually, poisoning is one of the leading causes of death in babies. Statistics show that 90% of these cases occur at home. But, we should not only focus on babies, as even older people can fall victim to poisoning.

There are some practices we tend to undermine, but have the capacity to end our life in one instant. In this chapter, we will look at ways you can take to reduce the occurrence of poisoning accidents.

- ***Keep Medicine Unreachable to Children***: Kids are good at eating everything they find. For this reason, poisoning from medicine is something you should look out for. The same goes for makeup, pesticides, and plants. If you cannot move the harmful product somewhere safe, block the way leading to that place.

- ***Have Child Safety Locks***: Locking places that house harmful products with child safety locks is a great way of reducing the risk.

- ***Keep Products in Original Containers***: You might forget or someone might use it thinking it is something else. If you do not have any other option, label it clearly.

- ***Keep Household Items and Food Separate***: It goes in the same lines that someone might just show up and use that product thinking it is food.

- ***Use Child Resistant Packages***: You might also consider in investing in child-resistant packages for medicine and other harmful products.

- ***Do not Call Medicine Candy***: Some have a tendency of calling medicine candy when giving it to kids. But this is wrong as the child might reach for the medicine and take it while you are away.

- ***Wash Hands Before Preparing Food***: Our hands come into contact with a lot of things and touching food before washing them might contaminate the food.

- ***Watch Expiry Dates***: Before eating food, always make sure that it is still good to be consumed. Many cases of food poisoning are a result of eating expired food.

- ***Keep Food in Containers***: Food should be kept in containers that have lids. Insects and other organisms might easily contaminate it if you just leave it in the open.

- ***Install Carbon Monoxide Alarms***: One of the leading causes of poisoning in adults at home is carbon monoxide. Making it even worse, you never see or smell it - hence being called the silent killer. But with a CO alarm, you can easily detect it before it kills you.

Chapter # 4: Reduce the Risk of Drowning

Spending time in the water is definitely a good time waster, especially during the summer. It should not be surprising to note that drowning happens to be the second leading cause of unintentional injury death. But, it is not always at the beach where there is a risk of drowning – it can even happen at home with just an inch of water.

To make matters worse, it is not always easy to know when someone is drowning. Forget about the victim screaming for help, as in most cases, the head will be under water, rendering the ability to speak impossible.

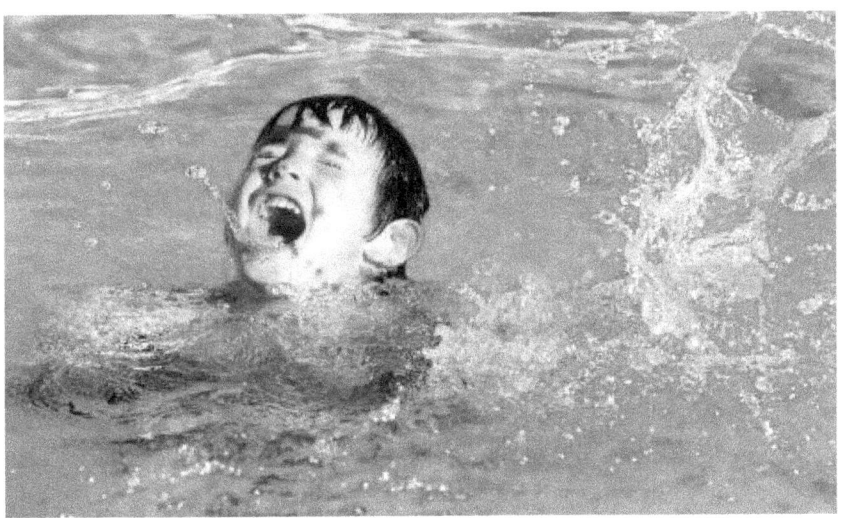

Although not all drowning accidents result in death, the non-fatal ones are enough to cause permanent brain damage. This can happen in pools, bathtubs, and even buckets of water. Children under the age of 5 are at the highest risk of drowning at home.

So without further ado, here are the steps you can take to secure your home from drowning accidents.

- ***Teach Children To Swim***: Having your kids learn how to swim at an early age will increase their chances of surviving if they ever come face to face with drowning. But that should not give you a peace of mind, as a young swimmer is still more vulnerable than an older child with no swimming skills.

- ***Install a Barrier Around the Pool***: Having a fence greatly reduces the probability of drowning by kids. However, for adults, a fence is not of much help. It is advised to build a four-sided fence with a gate that is unreachable to children. If dealing with an above ground pool, consider removing the ladders. Additionally, covering the pool is also a great barrier.

- ***Remove Toys From the Pool***: When done swimming, always remove any toys, as these can tempt children into getting back in the pool.

- ***Supervise Children***: Never leave children to swim in pools without adult supervision. This also applies to bathtubs or any buckets of water. For instance, if you are going to answer a call, wrap your child in a towel and bring them with you.

- ***Empty Buckets and Bathtubs***: Never leave buckets or bathtubs filled with water for no good reason. If you have to, close all doors that lead to these places.

- ***Take Showers***: Those who usually have seizures are advised to go for a shower instead of using the bathtub. It is easy to drown and die if you have a condition like epilepsy, in a bathtub.

- ***Learn CPR***: Knowing how to do CPR (Cardiopulmonary Resuscitation) might save someone who was about to drown. It only takes a few hours to master CPR and you can do it online.

- ***Never Swim When Drunk***: It might seem fun, going in water when drunk, but many have died as a result. So avoid it at all costs.

Chapter # 5: Keeping Wild Animals Away

Finding a large snake in your yard or a squirrel hiding in the chimney is probably the last thing you would want. The expansion of our residential areas has resulted in wild animals seeking shelter in our homes. Adding to this, we are a good source of food at times.

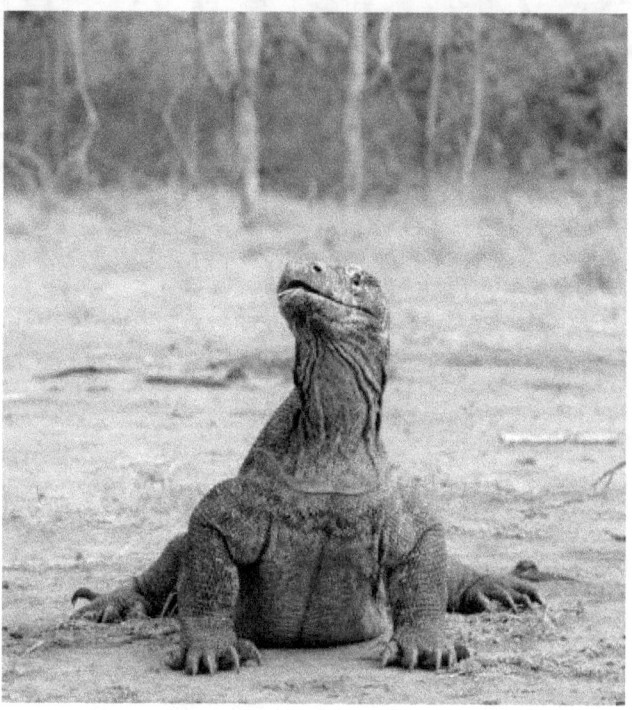

It is fun to watch wild animals, but not in your yard – only on TV. So this chapter will focus on ways you can take to reduce the likelihood of animals helping themselves into your home.

Here are some steps to take:

- ***Inspect Your House***: It is always amazing how you might miss a hole leading into your house, only to realize its presence when mice, raccoons, or other animals have made good use of it. So start by looking around your house for any holes. If you find one, seal it before some wild animal makes a village out of it.

- **Clean the Chimney**: Chimneys are known for harboring a lot of wild animals. If you have not used it in a while, inspect it before starting a fire, as it could be housing families. If in doubt, hire a professional to clean it for you.

- **Clear Vegetation**: Vegetation definitely makes the yard look attractive. However, you must understand that there is a fine line between an attractive yard and a perfect shelter for wild animals like snakes and other small mammals. If there are always people in this area, then it could be a dangerous situation.

- **Get Rid of Rocks**: If you have some big rocks on your yard, it is a better idea to get rid of them. Just like with vegetation, these also provide good cover to snakes and other animals. Additionally, they could provide shelter to animals that might be prey to other dangerous animals.

- **Do Not Keep Wood On The Ground**: Wood is another popular place for animals to hide and putting it on the ground increases the risk. So if you can, keep it somewhere elevated.

- **Close Garbage Cans**: Since food is one thing animals can't keep off their mind, it is not surprising that garbage cans happen to be their best friend. So make sure yours has a tight fitting lid and that you close it all the time, even when empty. You might also consider putting a weight on top.

- **Install a Fence**: Having a fence is another simple and effective way of keeping animals away. Areas under open porches or decks should be enclosed with wire mesh.

- **Close Doors**: Closing doors in your house all the time will keep animals from moving room to room.

- **Install Lights**: This works in two ways; it provides a way for you to see all around the yard when it is dark and it makes wild animals feel they are not in their natural habitat.

- **Get a Dog or Cat**: These two animals are great to keep as pets, but at the same time, they will help you know when the yard has been invaded by a wild animal. For example, a dog will most likely bark.

Chapter # 6: Minimizing the Risk of Electrocution

It is probably because we live with electricity daily that makes us take it for granted. However, there is a price to pay if you do not follow the rules. Electrocution can occur to anyone at any time and has the ability to damage our muscles and even internal organs like the brain, kidneys, etc.

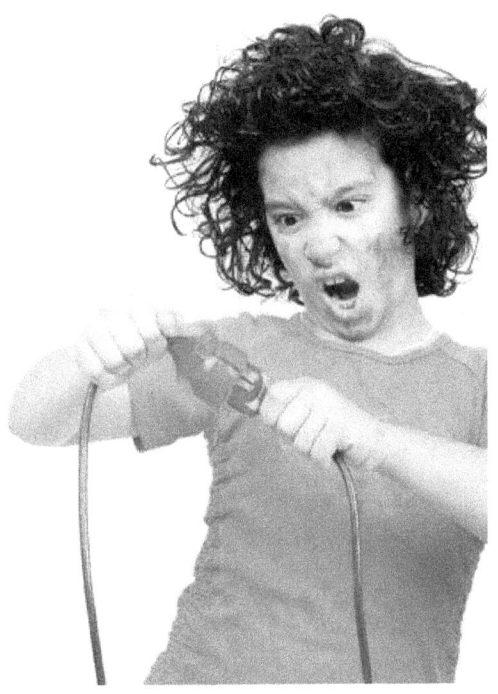

In some instances, it can disrupt breathing and stop the heart, which can lead to death. Each year, thousands die as a result of electrocution and thousands more are treated with electricity-related injuries.

Here is what you can do to remove this danger from your home:

- ***Replace Damaged Cords***: Any cord that exposes its wires is a disaster waiting to happen. The human body is a good conductor of electricity, and you will get electrocuted if you come in contact with such wires. This could be on an electrical appliance, extension cord, etc.

- *Hire a Professional*: Watching someone repair electrical appliances makes it look easy. And because of this, many have fallen in the trap of repairing their appliances themselves. If you have never had a chance to learn how to work with electricity, avoid this and hire a professional.

- *Do Not Use Extension Cords Permanently*: This is one thing many people ignore. However, you can avoid this by having more sockets installed in your home.

- *Do Not Overload Sockets*: Overloading a socket can easily burn off its insulation and start a fire. But most importantly, it increases your chances of getting electrocuted.

- *Replace Damaged Appliances*: Using a damaged electrical appliance is also one thing many do from time to time. But this should not be the case. If you cannot get it repaired, you should consider buying something new.

- *Do Not Use Electricity Near Water*: Water and electricity do not go together. If you are wet, you should never think of touching an electrical appliance. Again, you should never use an electrical appliance that is wet.

- *Do Not Pull The Cord*: Some have a tendency of removing appliances from the socket by pulling the cord. But this is very dangerous – instead, remove by pulling the plug.

- *Avoid Using Electricity During Thunderstorms*: When there is a thunderstorm, you should avoid using electrical appliances which could include laptops, iron, hair dryer, etc. These are known to attract lighting with enough power to kill a person instantly.

- *Inspect Pools and Hot Tubs*: Improper or damaged wiring in pools or hot tubs is known to claim a lot of lives, though we often overlook it. Call a professional to inspect yours, especially if it is old.

- *Cover Sockets*: Covering a socket will prevent children from inserting fingers or metal objects which could end up in electrocution.

Chapter # 7: Secure the Garden

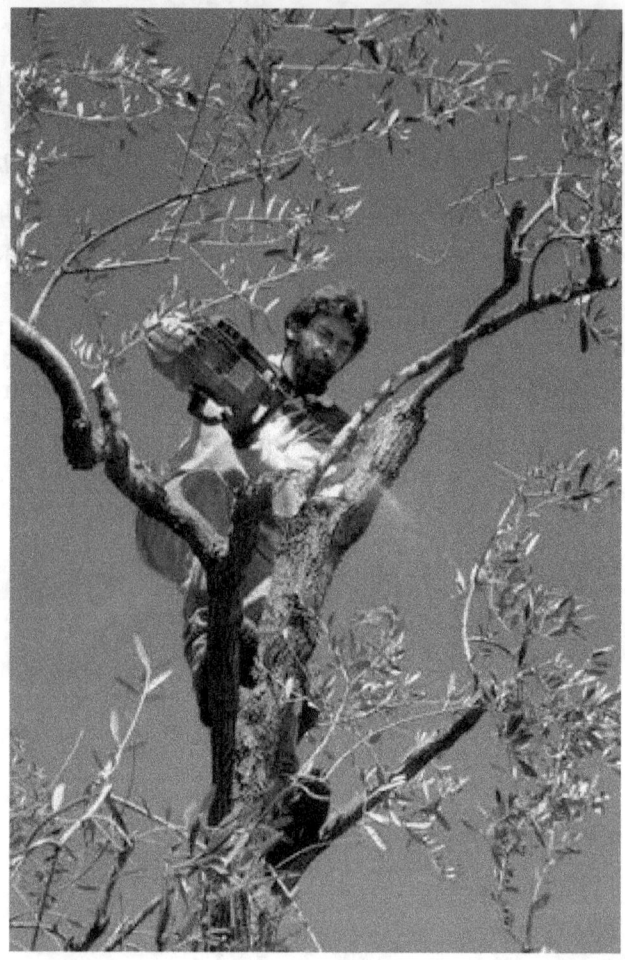

A home garden provides the perfect environment to hang out and have fun with family and friends. However, this sanctuary is not devoid of accidents. Time and again, people get hurt, especially kids, and in some situations, the results are fatal. But that should not scare you into giving up on your dreams of owning a home garden. There are some things you can do to make it safe.

While much of what will be said in this chapter will seem obvious to many, these are the things that are still often overlooked. Here are the tips:

- **Keep Tools Safely**: If you are working in the lawn, for example, with sharp tools, it is easy to just throw these on the ground. However, this is dangerous and you are advised to put them down safely with the sharp side facing down. And when you are done, lock these immediately.

- **Avoid Using Electric Appliances in Wet Weather**: If the ground is wet, you should avoid using electric appliances (e.g. lawn mower) or you will end up getting electrocuted.

- **Wear Protective Clothes**: You should also invest in protective clothing, which could include gloves, earplugs, work boots, and goggles. Additionally, you should tuck in your shirt at all times when working in the garden.

- **Do Not Plant Poisonous Plants**: Kids love playing in the garden and are notorious for tasting everything that raises their curiosity. So, to avoid the potential of poisoning, resist from planting poisonous plants, no matter how beautiful they may be. Otherwise, keep these away from children. Not only that, you should also teach them about the dangers of eating such plants as soon as they are old enough to make sense of what you are telling them.

- **Hide Pesticides**: The same goes for pesticides and other chemicals - keep these where children cannot reach them.

- **Never Leave Barbecue Unattended**: Doing this increases the risk of a fire. And when going away or to bed, double-check that you have indeed extinguished it.

- **Use Ladders Safely**: Many of the accidents in the garden are a result of a fall. If you are using a ladder, make sure it is in good condition.

Having rubber feet will also help keep it from slipping on the ground. You should also remember to never lean sideways, overstretch, or climb way too high – you will increase your chances of falling.

- ***Reduce Risk of Tripping***: If there is an uneven surface, pipes in the ground, or anything that might trip a person, remove these dangers early on.

- ***Call a Professional***: If you are unsure about doing something yourself, trust your instincts and avoid going DIY. Rather, hire a professional.

Chapter # 8: Protect Your Home from Storms

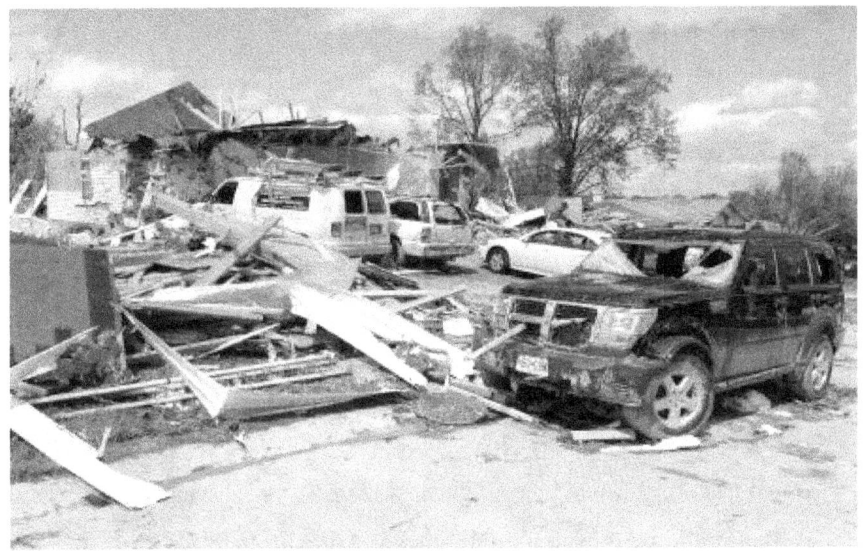

While coastal areas are among the best places on earth, they are also very susceptible to storms. We are lucky now as we are usually notified of impending storms well in time to get away. However, it's our homes and belongings that are left at the mercy of these disasters.

But, with a few tips, you might reduce the impact a storm can have on your house. Here they are:

- *Secure Windows*: Many believe the roof is the most venerable part during a storm, but this is not necessarily so, as a broken window can open Pandora's Box. If a window is smashed, wind will rush in and build enough pressure to lift the roof off and bring the walls down. Now many spend their energy tapping the windows to prevent this. But this is time wasting as tape does nothing in a storm. Instead, go for impact resistant windows. If that is not an option, you can cover them with plywood.

- ***Secure Garage Doors***: Same as with windows, garage doors are easily taken out in a storm because of their shape, and this can also result in the roof being blown away. As a prevention strategy, keep your car against the garage door to prevent it from barging in.

- ***Check the Roof for Damage***: From openings to unsecured tiles, a damaged roof increases the risk of destruction in a storm. For example, tiles might become projectiles and injure someone or break a window. So, fix these in advance.

- ***No Loose Items Around***: This could include pots in the garden, trampolines, bikes and anything that could easily be taken in a storm – these items must be brought inside or they risk becoming missiles that could land in somebody's head. And since storms know no boundaries, pay attention to your neighbor's home for anything that could end up in your house.

- ***Remove Overgrown Trees***: It does not matter if it was planted by your great grandfather, if a tree is too old with branches reaching for the house, then it is high time you give it a trim. Apparently, it is such trees that cause heavy destruction during storms.

- ***Stay Away From Windows***: If you fail to escape a storm, you should stay in your house and away from the windows. You can hide behind furniture or a sofa if you believe the windows will be smashed.

Chapter # 9: Protect Your Home From Burglary

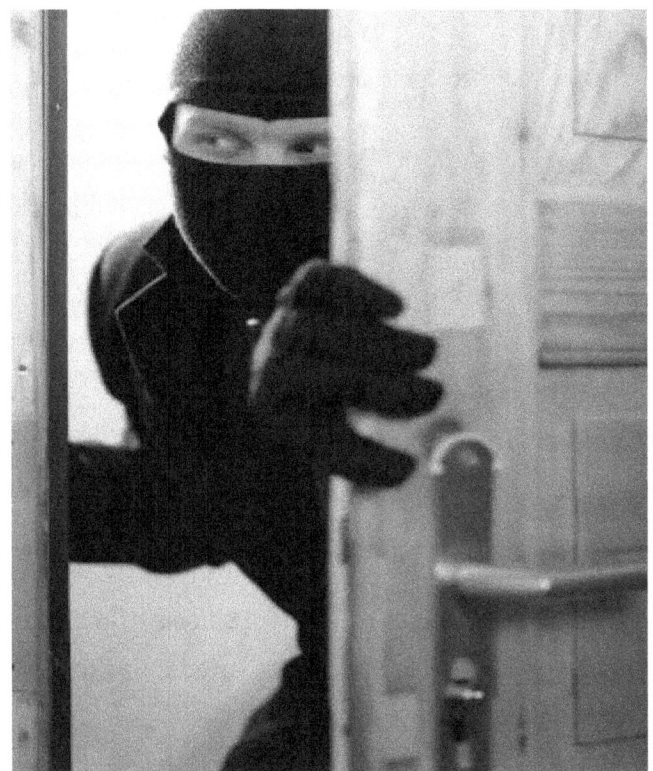

Being a victim of burglary can be a traumatizing experience, and with some people, it can take months to heal from such incidences both financially and emotionally. Even though you cannot secure your house 100%, there are things you can do to make it the last place a thief would think of robbing.

So without wasting any more time, here is what you can do:

- ***Pretend You Are Not Away***: Thieves are opportunists and like their work as easy as possible. That is why most of the break-ins occur when the owner is away. But that does not mean you should start working from home or cancel your holiday trips. Rather, eliminate things that show you are not at home. For example, if you will be gone for days, talk to a neighbor and ask them to park in your driveway or collect your mail. You can also arrange with someone to mow you lawn. Not only that, but you can use timers as well to turn on the radio or lights at random intervals.

- ***Invest in a Home Alarm System***: Having this will make thieves think twice before entering your home. The good thing is some are really cheap so owning one is not such a big deal.

- ***Lock Tools***: Thieves can also use your own tools like a ladder, hammer, ax, or other equipment to rob you. The problem is most people leave these in the yard or shed. However, locking them would eliminate the threat.

- ***Lock Doors and Windows***: As simple as this may sound, a good proportion of robberies are a result of unlocked doors and windows. So as a precaution, always lock these, even if you will be gone for only a few seconds.

- ***Have A Dog***: A barking dog is one of the simplest things you can use to know when an intruder comes near your house. It has also been discovered that simply having a "Beware of Dog" sign scares the devil out of most thieves.

- ***Clear Your Yard***: Going green is definitely a good thing for the environment. But at the same time, this presents a security risk – thieves use trees, bushes, or any kind of vegetation as cover. So trim these or you risk being the next victim of a burglary.

- ***Have A Safe***: Jewelry and other valuables are a thieves best bet, but investing in a small safe would be all you need to secure these.

- ***Know Your Neighbors***: Knowing who lives in the house next to yours can be very beneficial. It makes it easy to notify the police for any strangers in your house.

- ***Make Your House Number Visible***: Having your house number clearly visible both during day and night will make finding your house easy and fast during an emergency.

- ***Don't Talk About Your Trips in Public***: If you will be going away, share this with only those you can trust. Avoid posting on social networks, as thieves could be watching you.

- ***Hide Keys in Safe Places***: Keeping spare keys under flowers or similar places is something many do from time to time. Unfortunately, thieves are well aware of this. If you cannot find a not so obvious place to hide yours, entrust them to a friend who lives nearby. You can always call them if you lose your main keys.

Chapter # 10: Minimizing the Damage From Floods

If only we had wings and could fly, perhaps we would not be so concerned with floods. And with trends showing an increase in this disaster, we can only hope for the best. Partly, global warming is to blame for this as warmer air holds more water leading to more precipitation.

While there is no way of completely avoiding a flood, there are some steps you can take to minimize its damage. Here is what you can do:

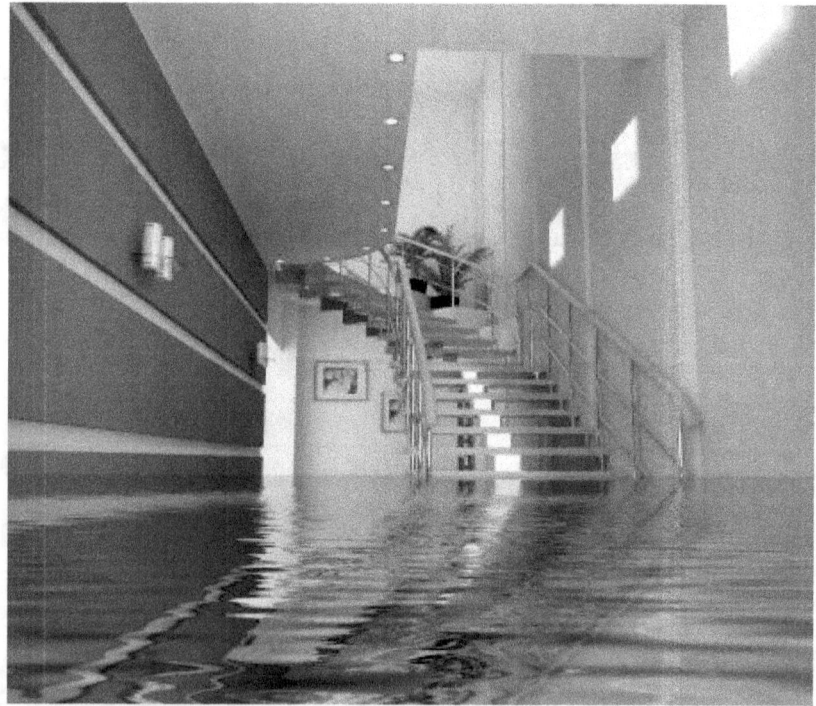

- ***Raise Sockets***: The one and only best way of avoiding a flood is elevation. Since water and electricity can lead to electrocution, you should have your sockets installed at least 1.5 meters from the ground. Usually, most floods do not get to that level, and as a precaution, avoiding using electric appliances that are wet.

- *Move Your Belongings*: All your electric appliances and any item that might be damaged by floods should be moved to upper floors in you have a multi-story house.

- *Cover Air Bricks*: Airbricks usually let in more of water to houses than you can imagine. To avoid this, purchase anti-flood airbrick covers.

- *Purchase Door Flood Barriers*: As with air bricks, water will also find its way into your house through the door. Therefore, you should purchase a flood barrier. If the water level is not that high, you might also consider using sand bags.

- *Clear Gutters and Drains*: These will help take the water away, but if they are blocked, your worst fear will come to life before your very eyes.

- *Invest in a Pump*: You will need this to pump out all the water in your house. But since electricity is usually unavailable when a flood hits, you will be better off investing in a battery-powered pump.

- *Prevent Sewer Flooding*: This is one of the nastiest things that come with almost every flood. Thankfully, some great minds have invented valves that only allow sewage to flow in one direction.

- *Listen to The Authorities*: Most importantly, if you are advised to evacuate the area, do so as soon as possible. Your life is more important than the possessions you have in your home. This means you need to keep a close ear to the radio for disasters that are likely to hit where you live.

Conclusion

Having reached this far, I believe you have learned some tips you can employ to secure your house. You might think that this is simply being paranoid, only to realize that your home is not as safe as you thought when danger starts knocking on your door. Of course, sometimes it is a matter of being at the wrong place at the wrong time.

Home should be a paradise and not a place that keeps you awake all night, fearing for what might happen. Needless to say, it is also a place you share with those you care about most. So taking the time to reduce the risks likely to occur is your way of showing these people that you care. It may never come close to how secure the white house is, but like the old saying goes, little is better than nothing.

Author Bio

Muhammad Usman is a distinguished medical graduate of Allama Iqbal medical college (AIMC). He is a professional writer who has been in the field for more than 4 years. During this time he has produced 10,000+ articles, blogs and eBooks on various niches related to diseases, health, fitness, nutrition and well-being. He is a regular contributor to several journals related to medicine and surgery. He is the editor of several journals and newspapers.

Check out some of the other JD-Biz Publishing books
Gardening Series on Amazon

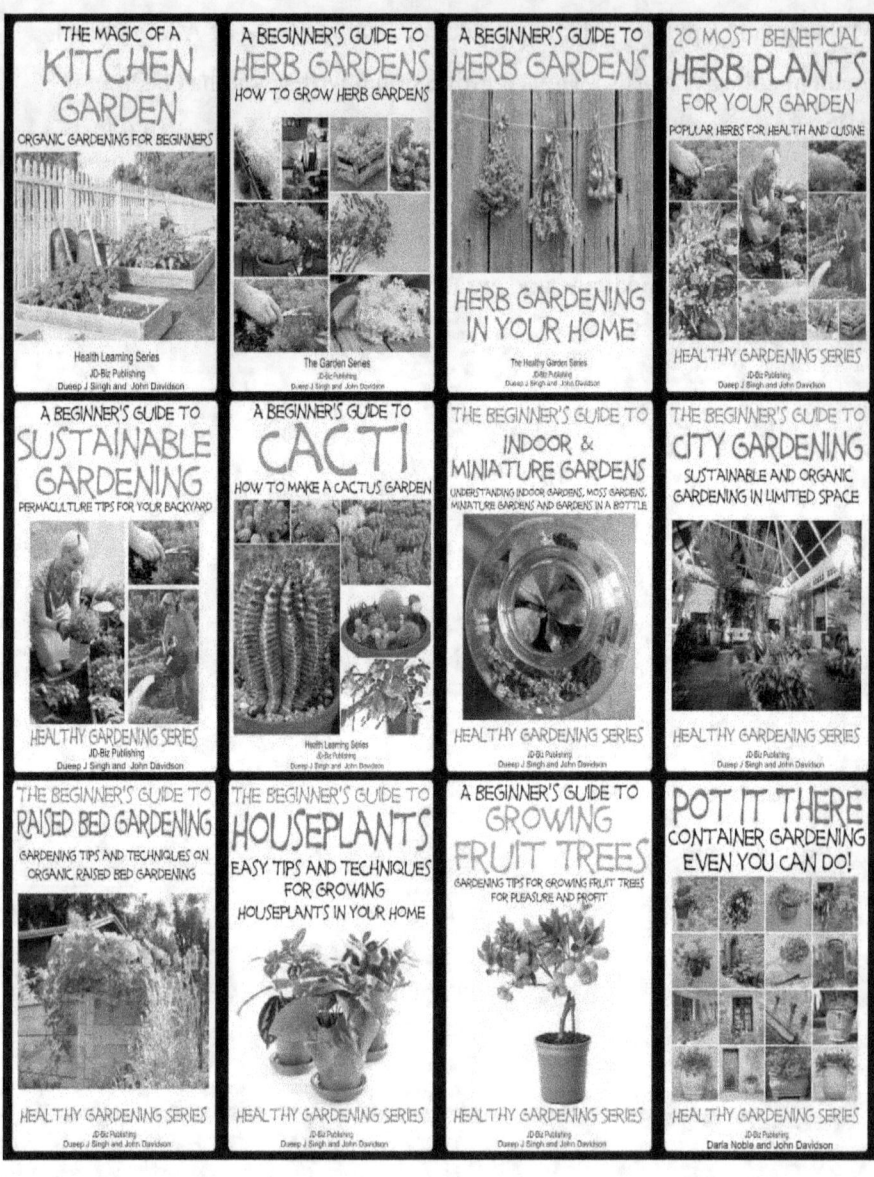

Health Learning Series

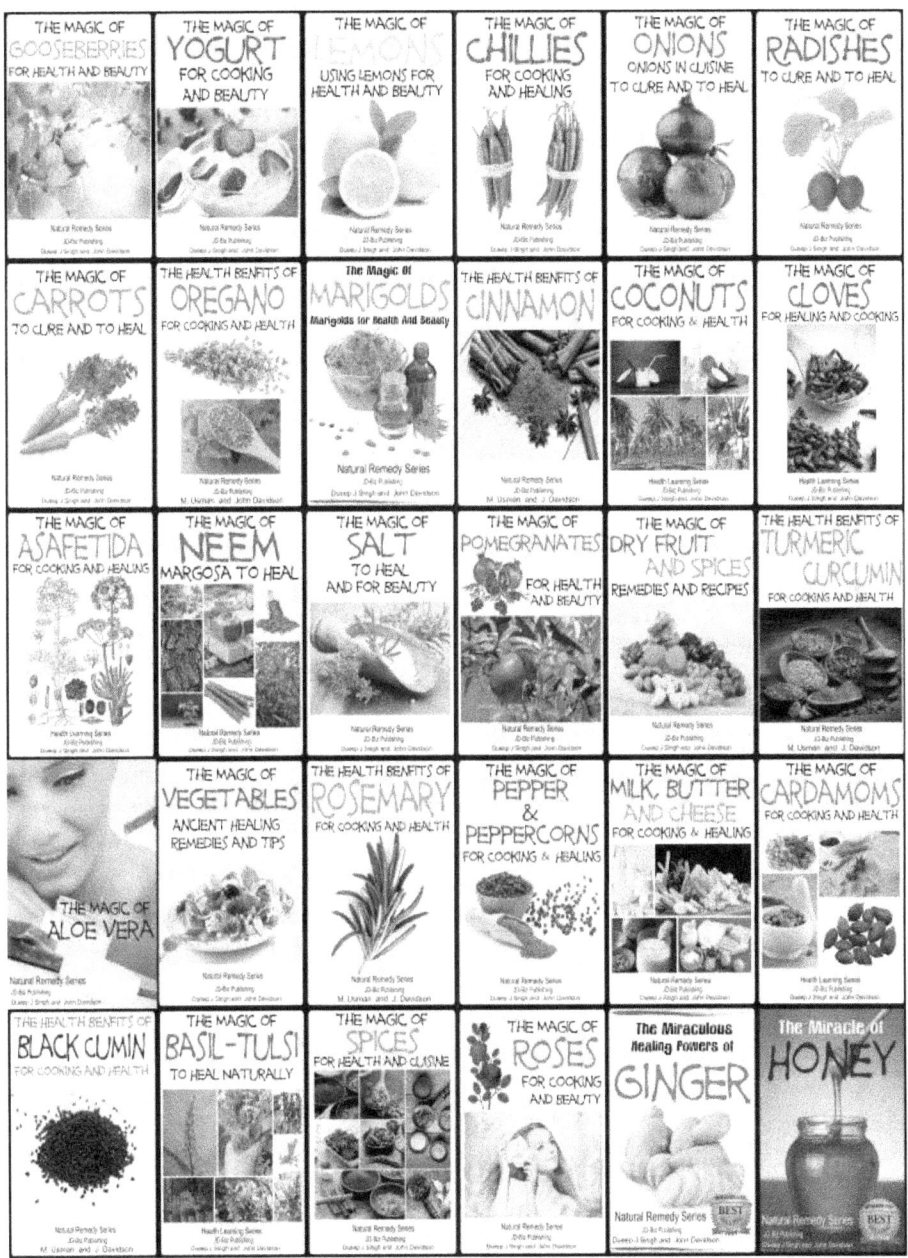

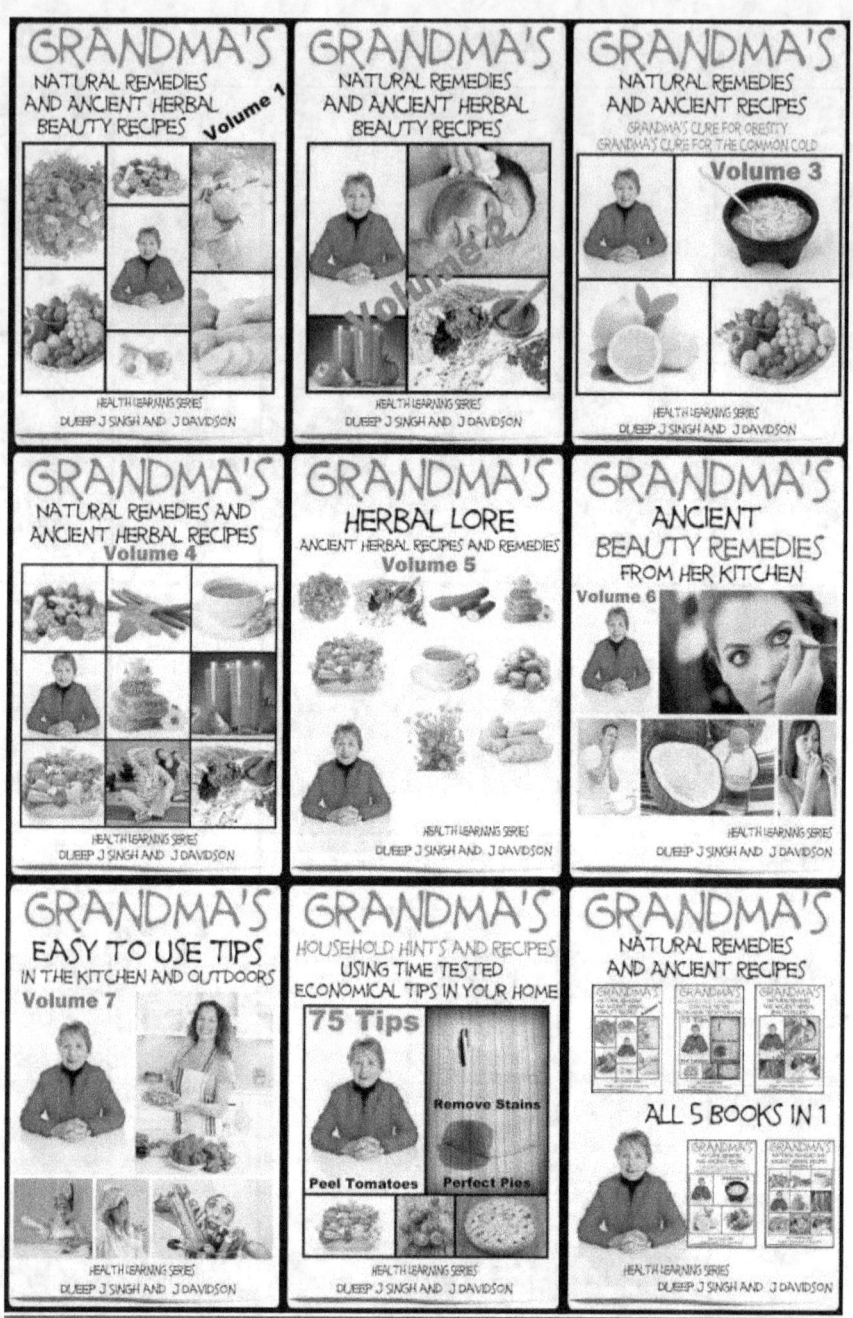

Country Life Books

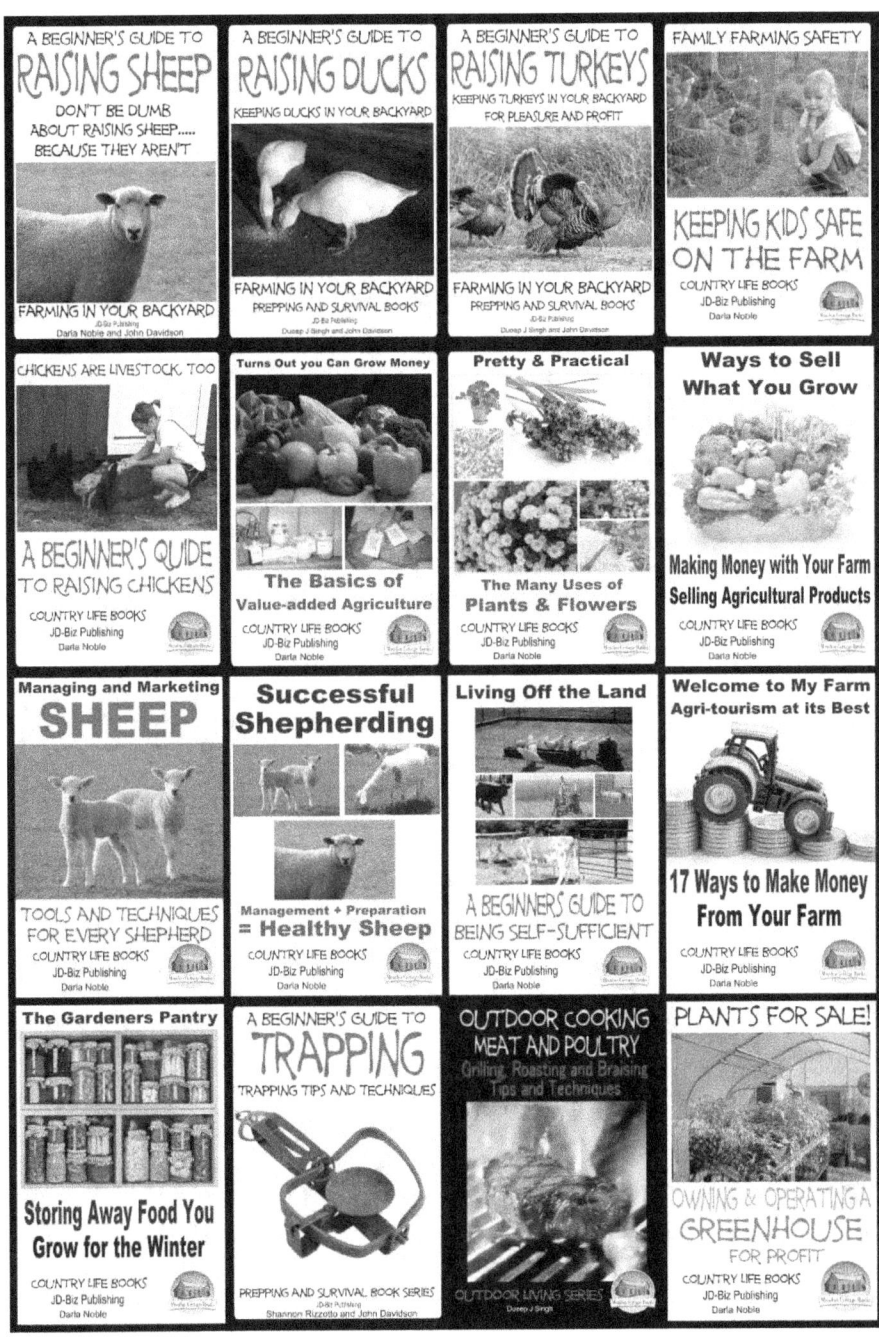

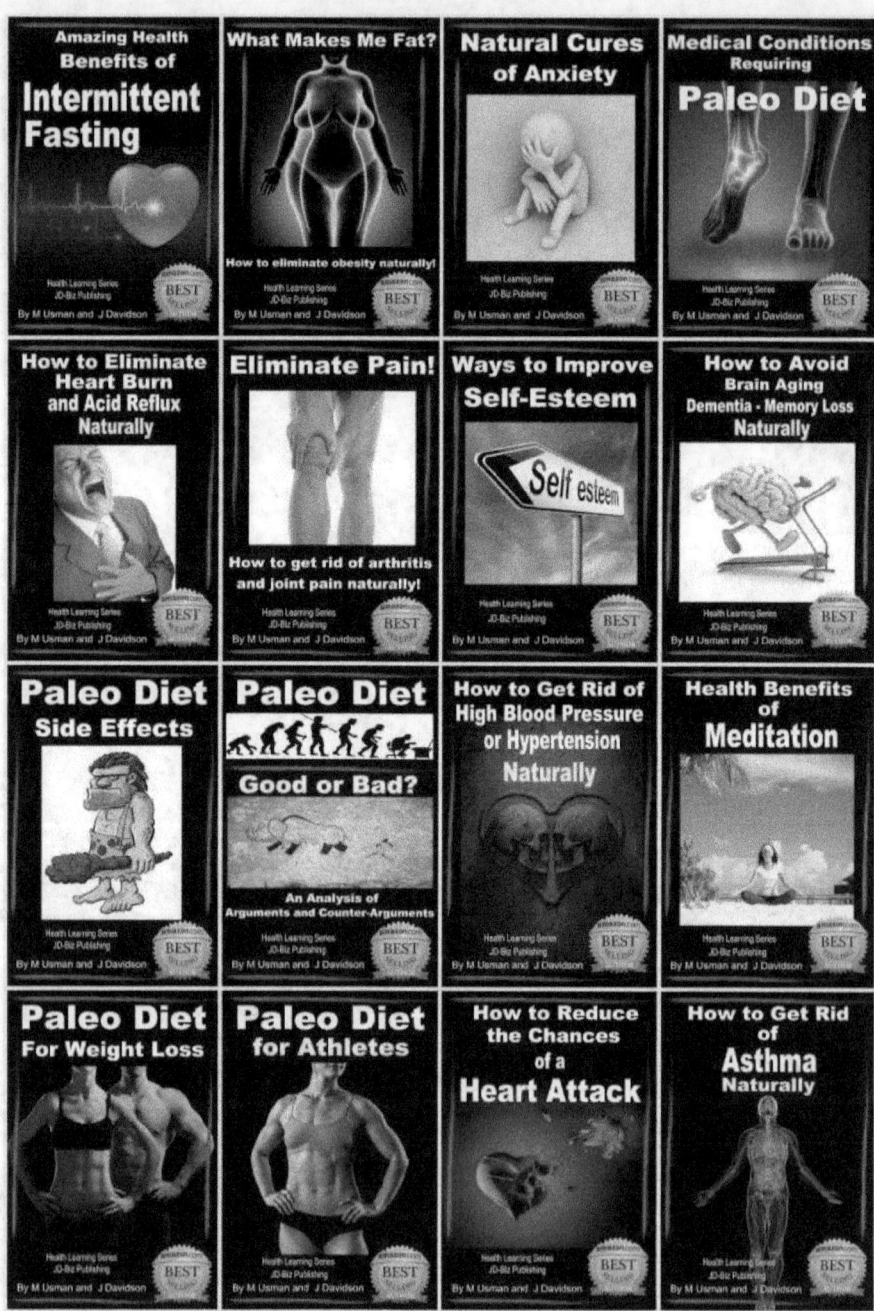

Amazing Animal Book Series

Learn To Draw Series

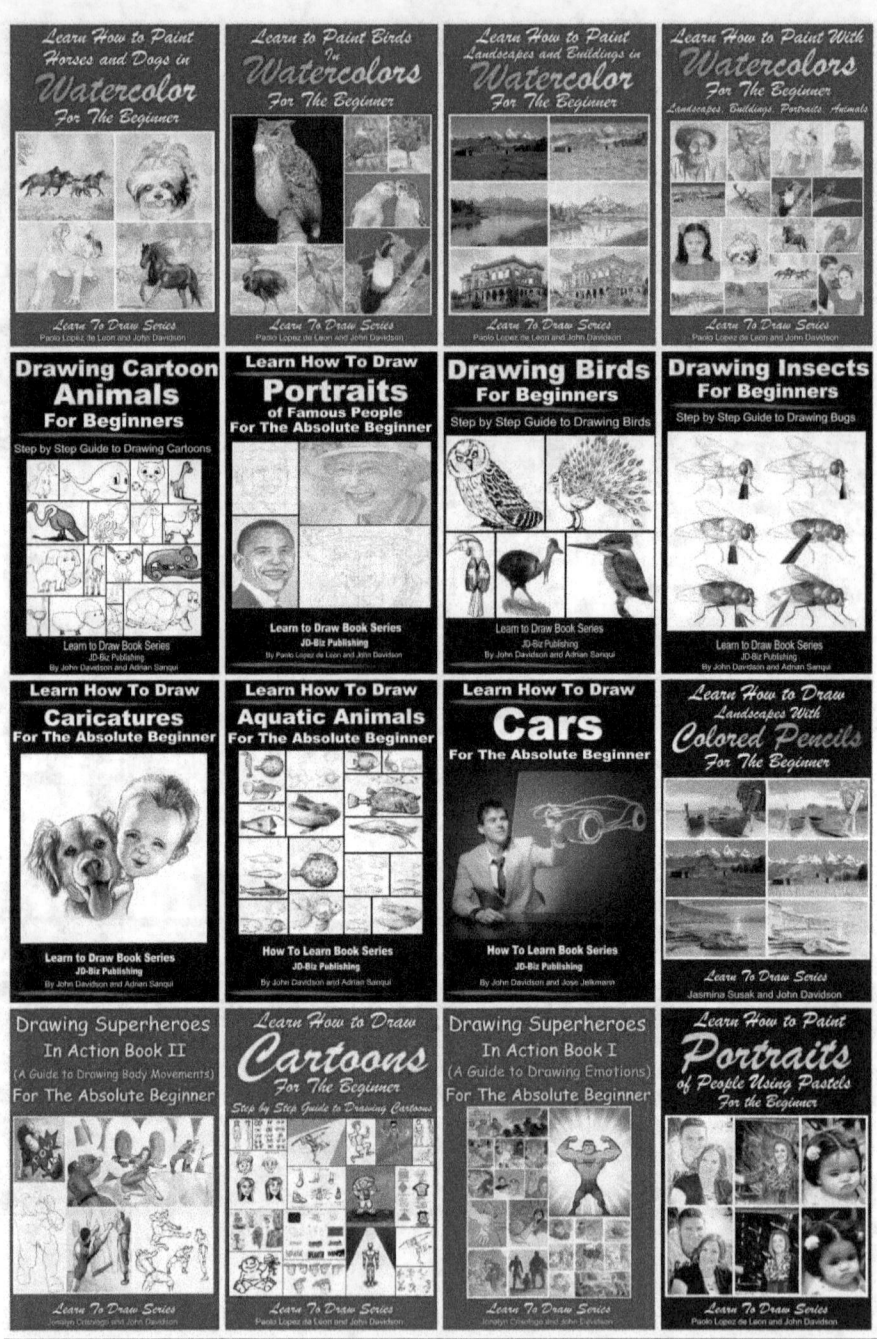

How to Build and Plan Books

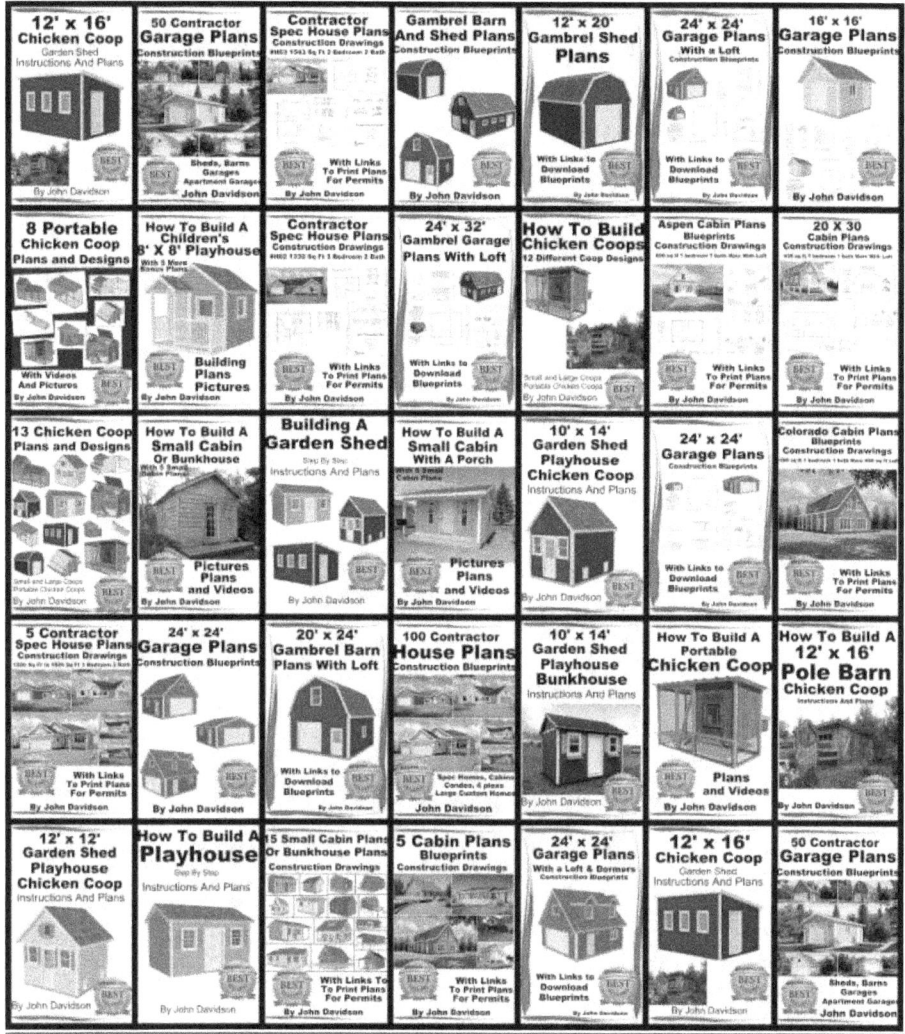

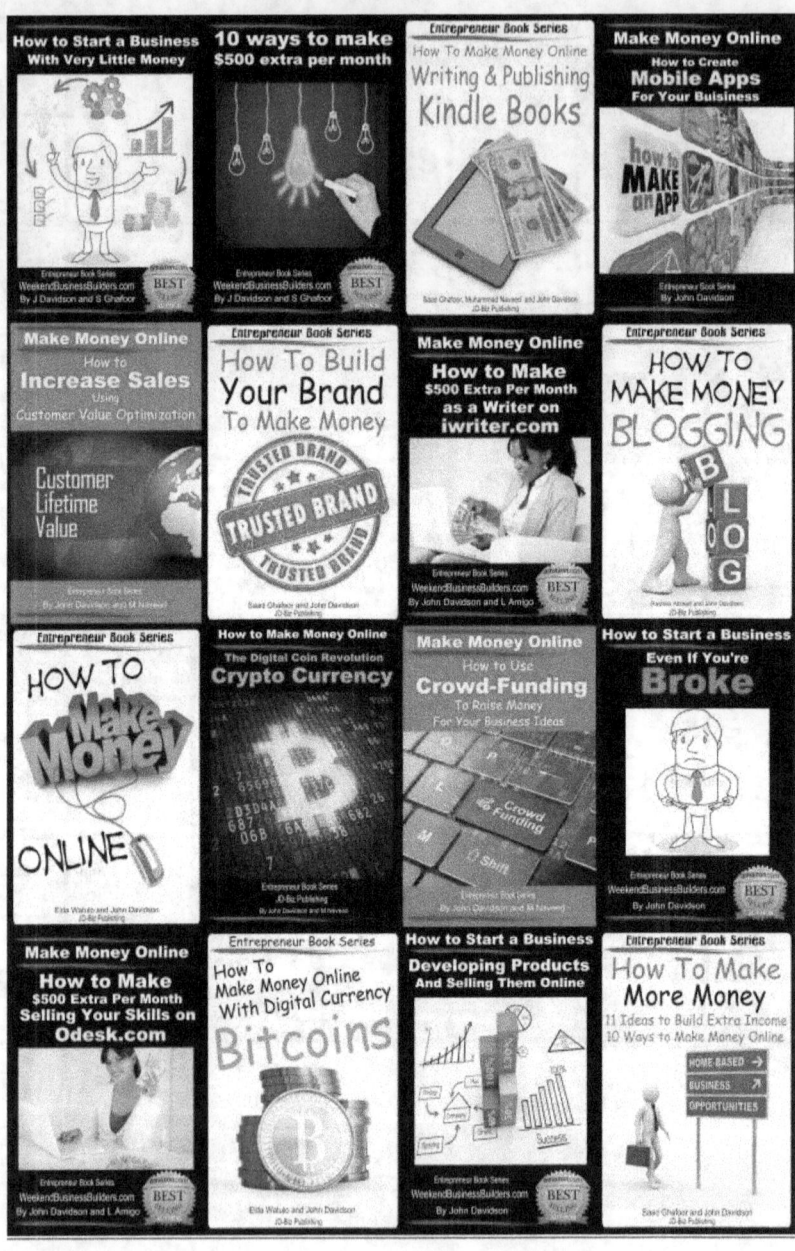

Our books are available at

1. Amazon.com

2. Barnes and Noble

3. Itunes

4. Kobo

5. Smashwords

6. Google Play Books

Publisher

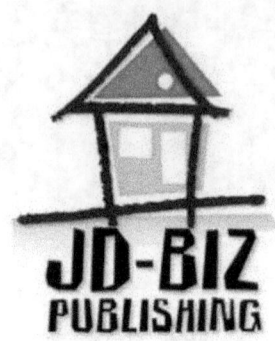

JD-Biz Corp

P O Box 374

Mendon, Utah 84325

http://www.jd-biz.com/

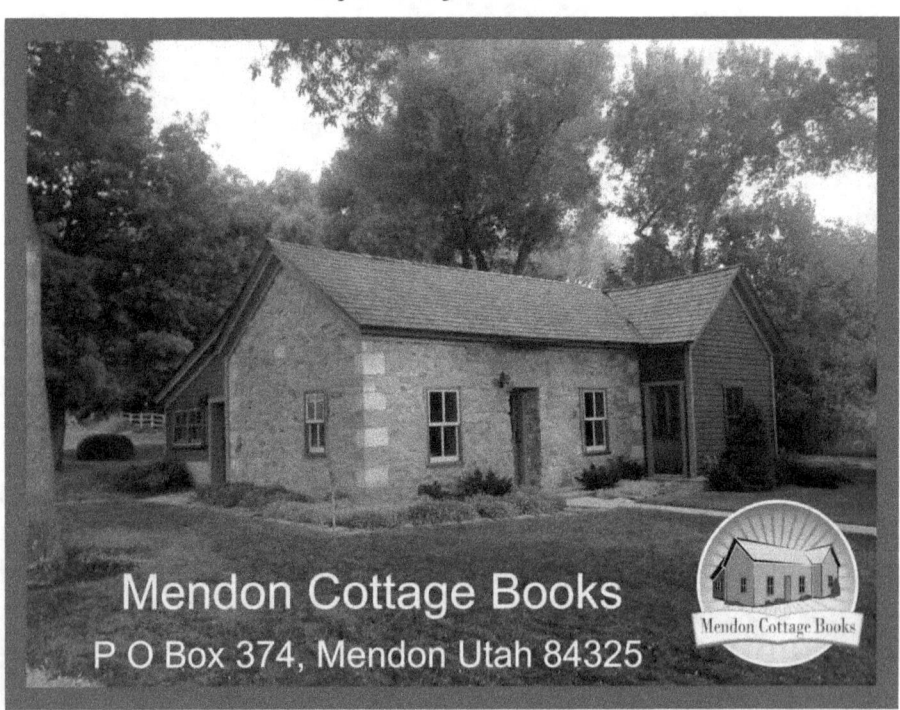

Mendon Cottage Books

P O Box 374, Mendon Utah 84325

www.ingramcontent.com/pod-product-compliance
Lightning Source LLC
Chambersburg PA
CBHW070841290526
45795CB00002B/939